C000179677

Keto Diet Cookbook for Beginners

-The Optimal Keto-Friendly Cookbook for Beginners -

[Dr. Dean Chasey]

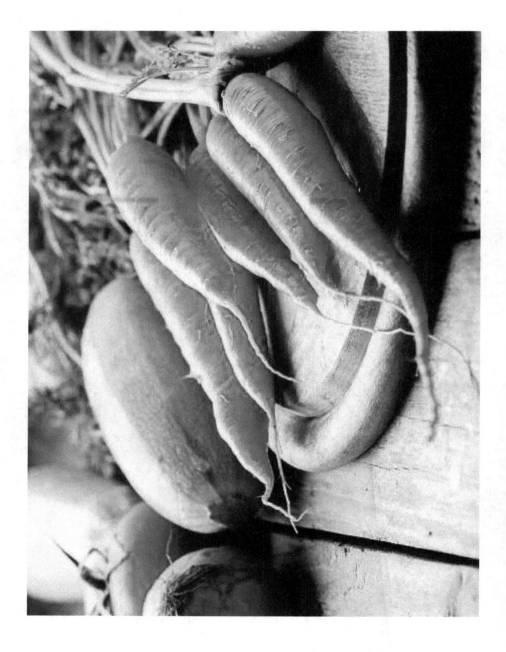

Table Of Content

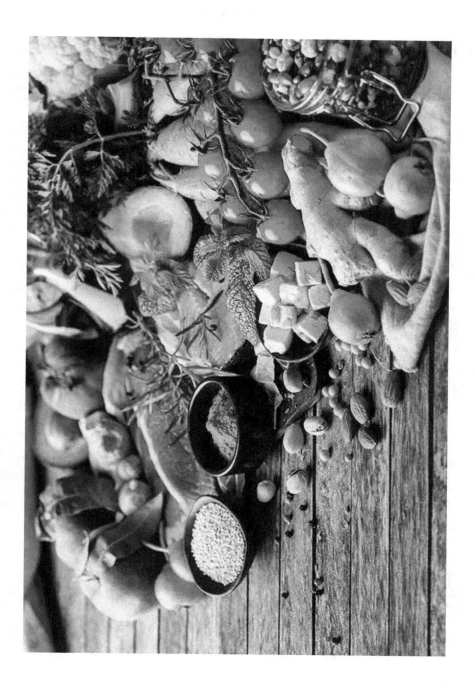

© Copyright 2020 by Dr. Dean Chasey All rights reserved.

The following Book is reproduced below with the goal of providing information that is as accurate and reliable as possible. Regardless, purchasing this Book can be seen as consent to the fact that both the publisher and the author of this book are in no way experts on the topics discussed within and that any recommendations or suggestions that are made herein are for entertainment purposes only. Professionals should be consulted as needed prior to undertaking any of the action endorsed herein.

This declaration is deemed fair and valid by both the American Bar Association and the Committee of Publishers Association and is legally binding throughout the United States.

Furthermore, the transmission, duplication, or reproduction of any of the following work including specific information will be considered an illegal act irrespective of if it is done electronically or in print. This extends to creating a secondary or tertiary copy of the work or a recorded copy and is only allowed with the express written consent from the Publisher. All additional right reserved.

The information in the following pages is broadly considered a truthful and accurate account of facts and as such, any inattention, use, or misuse of the information in question by the reader will render any resulting actions solely under their purview. There are no scenarios in which the publisher or the original author of this work can be in any fashion deemed liable for any hardship or damages that may befall them after undertaking information described herein.

Additionally, the information in the following pages is intended only for informational purposes and should thus be thought of as universal. As befitting its nature, it is presented without assurance regarding its prolonged validity or interim quality. Trademarks that are mentioned are done without written consent and can in no way be considered an endorsement from the trademark holder.

CHAPTER 1: **BREAKFAST**

Ginger Pancakes

Prep:

10 mins

Cook:

10 mins

Total:

20 mins

Servings:

8

Yield:

8 servings

Ingredients

1 ⅓ cups milk
cooking spray
1 egg
1 tablespoon applesauce
1 teaspoon vanilla extract
1 teaspoon ground cinnamon
2 teaspoons ground ginger
2 cups baking mix

Directions

1

Beat milk, egg, applesauce, ground ginger, vanilla extract, and cinnamon together in a bowl. Whisk baking mix into the milk mixture until just combined into a loose batter.

2

Prepare a skillet with cooking spray and place over medium heat.

3

Ladle about 1/4 cup batter into the prepared skillet; cook until bubbles begin to form on the top, 4 to 5 minutes. Turn the pancake and continue cooking until the other side of the pancake is golden brown, 3 to 5 minutes more. Transfer pancake to a plate and cover with a lid to keep warm. Repeat until batter is completely used.

Nutrition

Per Serving: 134 calories; protein 4.6g; carbohydrates 24.5g; fat 1.8g; cholesterol 23.7mg; sodium 601.8mg.

Bacon & Blue Cheese Cup

Prep:

10 mins

Additional:

1 hr

Total:

1 hr 10 mins

Servings:

10

Yield:

10 servings

Ingredients

½ cup blue cheese salad dressing

1 (2.5 ounce) package cooked real bacon pieces (such as Hormel™)

½ cup mayonnaise

1 (16 ounce) bag coleslaw mix

1 cup quartered cherry tomatoes

salt and pepper to taste

Directions

1

Combine mayonnaise, salad dressing, salt, and pepper in a large bowl. Stir in the coleslaw mix and bacon. Add the tomatoes, and toss gently. Cover, and refrigerate for 1 hour or overnight before serving.

Nutrition

Per Serving: 205 calories; protein 4.5g; carbohydrates 7.6g; fat 17.9g; cholesterol 15mg; sodium 434.6mg.

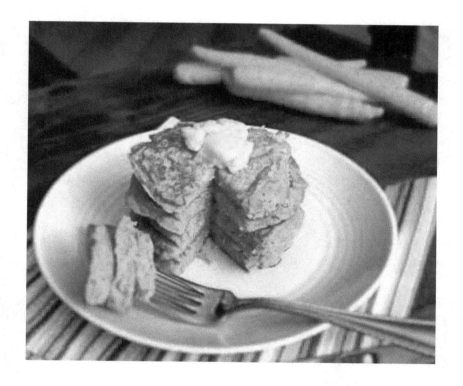

Acai Smoothie Bowl

Prep:

10 mins

Total:

10 mins

Servings:

2

Yield:

2 smoothie bowls

Ingredients

7 ounces frozen unsweetened acai pulp, partially defrosted in refrigerator overnight

1 cup blueberries

¾ cup almond milk, or more as needed

2 teaspoons honey

2 medium ripe frozen bananas

Topping:

1 medium banana, sliced

2 tablespoons fresh blueberries

1 tablespoon pomegranate seeds

1 tablespoon large coconut flakes

Directions

1

Combine acai, bananas, blueberries, almond milk, and honey in a blender. Blend until smooth. Smoothie should have a thick consistency, like frozen yogurt.

2

Pour into 2 bowls and top with banana slices, blueberries, pomegranate seeds, and coconut.

Nutrition

Per Serving: 347 calories; protein 3.3g; carbohydrates 68.1g; fat 8.7g; sodium 88.9mg.

Bacon & Cheese Frittata

Prep:

10 mins

Cook:

35 mins

Total:

45 mins

Servings:

6

Yield:

6 servings

Ingredients

5 slices bacon

1 cup shredded Cheddar cheese

6 eggs

1 cup milk

½ teaspoon salt

¼ teaspoon ground black pepper

¼ cup chopped green onions

2 tablespoons butter, melted

Directions

1

Preheat oven to 350 degrees F. Lightly grease a 7x11-inch baking dish.

2

Place bacon in a large skillet and cook over medium-high heat, turning occasionally, until evenly browned, about 10 minutes. Drain bacon slices on paper towels and crumble.

3

Beat eggs, milk, butter, salt, and ground pepper in a bowl; pour into prepared baking dish. Sprinkle with onions, bacon, and Cheddar cheese.

4

Bake in preheated oven until a knife inserted near the center comes out clean, 25 to 30 minutes.

Nutrition

Per Serving: 245 calories; protein 15.3g; carbohydrates 3g; fat 19.1g; cholesterol 227.6mg; sodium 602.5mg.

Walnut Granola

Servings:

20

Yield:

10 cups

Ingredients

2 bananas, peeled and diced

¼ cup packed brown sugar

¼ cup hot water

1 tablespoon vanilla extract

1 ¼ cups dates, pitted and chopped

1 teaspoon ground cinnamon

8 ounces dried mixed fruit

8 ounces blanched slivered almonds

8 cups quick cooking oats

Directions

1

Preheat oven to 250 degrees F.

2

Puree the bananas and dates in a food processor. Add the brown sugar, hot water, vanilla and cinnamon; mix well.

3

Pour mixture into a large mixing bowl, add oatmeal and mix well.

4

Spread onto large baking sheets and bake at 250 degrees Ffor 1 to 1 1/2 hours stirring frequently. Cook longer for crunchier if desired. Once cooled add the dried fruits and nuts, as little or as much as you want, and mix.

Nutrition

Per Serving: 267 calories; protein 7.2g; carbohydrates 43.8g; fat 7.9g; sodium 6.3mg.

Asparagus Omelet

Prep:

15 mins

Cook:

10 mins

Total:

25 mins

Servings:

2

Yield:

1 large omelet

Ingredients

3 tablespoons olive oil, or as needed

¼ cup chopped onion

1 pound ham steak, cut into small pieces

5 large eggs

4 asparagus spears, chopped

2 slices Provolone cheese

¼ cup chopped green pepper

1 teaspoon garlic salt

Directions

1

Heat olive oil in a pan over medium heat; add onion and green pepper. Cook and stir until onion is slightly brown, about 5 minutes. Stir in ham and garlic salt.

2

Beat eggs, asparagus, and milk together with a whisk or a fork in a bowl; pour over ham mixture. Add whole Provolone cheese slices or break them into pieces. Cook until eggs begin to set, about 3 minutes. Gently fold the omelet in half; cook until cheese melts, about 2 minutes.

Nutrition

Per Serving: 739 calories; protein 67.1g; carbohydrates 6.4g; fat 48.8g; cholesterol 531.9mg; sodium 4191.4mg.

Ricotta Cheese

Prep:

10 mins

Cook:

20 mins

Additional:

20 mins

Total:

50 mins

Servings:

16

Yield:

28 ounces ricotta cheese

Ingredients

¼ cup water
1 gallon raw milk
1 teaspoon citric acid powder

Directions

1

Combine water and citric acid in a small bowl; mix until dissolved.

2

Pour milk into a large pot set over medium heat. Heat milk, stirring occasionally, until it registers 185 degrees F on an instant-read thermometer. Do not boil and stir often to prevent scorching. Stir in citric acid. Keep stirring until curds form.

3

Scoop curds into a sieve lined with several layers of cheesecloth using a slotted spoon. Fold the edges of the cheesecloth over the curds and let drain over a bowl at room temperature, 20 to 30 minutes.

4

Remove the cheese from the cheesecloth and cream and salt. Stir well to combine. Serve right away as-is or use in your favorite recipe.

Nutrition

Per Serving: 153 calories; protein 7.9g; carbohydrates 11.2g; fat 8.6g; cholesterol 26.9mg; sodium 389.1mg.

Raspberry Mini Tarts

Prep:

1 hr 10 mins

Additional:

1 hr

Total:

2 hrs 10 mins

Servings:

8

Yield:

1 - 9 inch tart

Ingredients

1 cup all-purpose flour

½ cup butter

4 cups fresh raspberries

1 (8 ounce) jar raspberry jam

2 tablespoons confectioners' sugar

Directions

1

In a medium bowl, blend together the flour, butter and sugar. Chill mixture for 1 hour.

2

Preheat oven to 375 degrees F.

3

Pat chilled mixture into a 9 inch tart pan.

4

Bake in preheated oven for 10 minutes. Once out of the oven, allow to cool.

5

Arrange raspberries in crust. Heat jar of jam in microwave until it begins to boil. Pour jam over fruit. Cover and refrigerate tart for about 1 hour.

Nutrition

Per Serving: 266 calories; protein 2.3g; carbohydrates 39.1g; fat 12g; cholesterol 30.5mg; sodium 82.1mg.

Pecan Cookies

Prep:

20 mins

Cook:

10 mins

Total:

30 mins

Servings:

24

Yield:

2 dozen

Ingredients

1 teaspoon baking powder

9 tablespoons SPLENDA® Granular

¼ teaspoon baking soda

¼ teaspoon salt

½ cup butter or margarine

3 tablespoons brown sugar replacement (e.g. Sugar Twin)

1 egg, lightly beaten

½ teaspoon vanilla extract

1 ¼ cups all-purpose flour

1 cup chopped pecans

Directions

1

Preheat the oven to 375 degrees F. Sift together flour, baking powder, baking soda, and salt.

2

In a mixing bowl, cream together butter and sugar replacements. Beat in egg and vanilla. Mix in flour mixture. Stir in pecans. Drop by rounded teaspoon onto ungreased baking sheet.

3

Bake in preheated oven for about 10 minutes. Cool cookies slightly before removing from pan.

Nutrition

Per Serving: 93 calories; protein 1.4g; carbohydrates 5.8g; fat 7.4g; cholesterol 17.9mg; sodium 83.5mg.

Leck Lentil Soup

Servings:

6

Yield:

6 servings

Ingredients

1 onion, chopped

¼ cup olive oil

2 carrots, diced

2 stalks celery, chopped

1 teaspoon dried oregano

1 bay leaf

1 teaspoon dried basil

1 (14.5 ounce) can crushed tomatoes

2 cups dry lentils

2 cloves garlic, minced

8 cups water

2 tablespoons vinegar

salt to taste

½ cup spinach, rinsed and thinly sliced

ground black pepper to taste

Directions

1

In a large soup pot, heat oil over medium heat. Add onions, carrots, and celery; cook and stir until onion is tender. Stir in garlic, bay leaf, oregano, and basil; cook for 2 minutes.

2

Stir in lentils, and add water and tomatoes. Bring to a boil. Reduce heat, and simmer for at least 1 hour. When ready to serve stir in spinach, and cook until it wilts. Stir in vinegar, and season to taste with salt and pepper, and more vinegar if desired.

Nutrition

Per Serving: 349 calories; protein 18.3g; carbohydrates 48.2g; fat 10g; sodium 130.5mg.

Mushroom Frittata

Prep:

10 mins

Cook:

23 mins

Total:

33 mins

Servings:

4

Yield:

4 servings

Ingredients

1 tablespoon vegetable oil

1 ½ cups mushrooms, sliced

½ cup diced yellow onion

4 garlic cloves, sliced

1 pinch red pepper flakes

6 slices Farmland® Bacon, large dice

2 cups fresh spinach

6 eggs

1 cup shredded Gouda cheese

2 tablespoons milk

Directions

1

Preheat oven to 350 degrees F.

2

In medium nonstick pan, heat vegetable oil over medium heat.

3

Add bacon and cook until crispy. Transfer bacon to paper towel-lined plate and reserve. Keep bacon fat in pan.

4

To pan with bacon fat, add mushrooms and cook until well browned. Remove and reserve.

5

Add onions and cook until softened; add garlic and cook for additional 2 minutes.

6

Add red pepper flakes and spinach. Cook until spinach just starts to wilt.

7

Return bacon and mushrooms to spinach mixture and add eggs whisked with 2 tablespoons milk, stirring to combine. Pour mixture into ovenproof serving dishes.

8

Top with smoked Gouda and place in oven. Bake for 8 to 10 minutes, or until eggs are just set.

Nutrition

Per Serving: 378 calories; protein 23.7g; carbohydrates 6.3g; fat 28.5g; cholesterol 328.8mg; sodium 713.9mg.

CHAPTER 2: SOUPS & SALADS

Broccoli Cheddar Soup

Prep:

10 mins

Cook:

15 mins

Total:

25 mins

Servings:

6

Yield:

6 servings

Ingredients

1 tablespoon butter
¼ cup minced shallot
2 cups chicken broth, divided
2 ounces cream cheese, softened
½ cup heavy whipping cream
8 ounces shredded Cheddar cheese
1 teaspoon xanthan gum
½ teaspoon garlic granules
freshly ground black pepper to taste
6 ounces frozen broccoli rice

Directions

1

Melt butter in a saucepan over medium heat. Add shallots and cook, stirring occasionally, until caramelized, about 5 minutes.

2

Slowly pour in 1/2 cup chicken broth and stir to scrape up any bits of shallot. Add cream cheese and whisk to break up any lumps. Pour in remaining broth and whipping cream. Stir in Cheddar cheese, riced broccoli, and garlic granules. Simmer for 4 minutes.

3

Add xanthan gum and whisk continuously until soup is thickened, 2 to 3 minutes. Serve immediately with freshly ground black pepper.

Nutrition

Per Serving: 295 calories; protein 11.8g; carbohydrates 5.2g; fat 25.3g; cholesterol 84.4mg; sodium 720.5mg.

Shrimp Salad with Cauliflower

Prep:

5 mins

Cook:

20 mins

Additional:

15 mins

Total:

40 mins

Servings:

10

Yield:

10 servings

Ingredients

1 head cauliflower, thinly sliced

1 tablespoon minced pimento

1 pound shrimp - cooked, peeled, deveined and chilled

3 eggs

1 cup mayonnaise

¾ cup creamy Italian-style salad dressing

¾ cup sliced black olives

1 cup chopped green onions

Directions

1

Place eggs in a small saucepan, and add water to cover. Cover the pan, and bring to a boil over high heat. Remove from heat and let stand covered for 12 minutes. Cool, peel, and chop the hard boiled eggs.

2

Mix mayonnaise and salad dressing together in a small bowl.

3

To a large bowl, add cauliflower, shrimp, green onions, chopped eggs, olives, and pimientos. Toss to combine. Stir in dressing mixture, and toss to coat. Refrigerate. Serve chilled.

Nutrition

Per Serving: 331 calories; protein 14.9g; carbohydrates 6.6g; fat 27.8g; cholesterol 156mg; sodium 542mg.

Chicken Vegetable Soup

Prep:

15 mins

Cook:

1 hr 15 mins

Total:

1 hr 30 mins

Servings:

4

Yield:

4 servings

Ingredients

1 cup chicken broth

1 cup chopped carrot

4 potatoes, cubed

1 (15 ounce) can green beans

¼ cup chopped green bell pepper

1 cup tomato juice

1 cup shredded cabbage

3 cloves garlic, minced

½ onion, chopped

½ teaspoon dried oregano

1 tablespoon dried basil

1 cup cooked and cubed chicken

½ teaspoon Italian-style seasoning

salt and pepper to taste

Directions

1

In a large pot over high heat, combine the chicken broth, cabbage, carrots, potatoes, onion, green beans, green bell pepper, tomato juice, garlic, oregano, basil and Italian-style seasoning.

2

Bring to a boil, reduce heat to low and simmer for 1 hour, or until all vegetables are tender.

3

Add the chicken and simmer for 15 more minutes. Season with salt and pepper to taste.

Nutrition

Per Serving: 317 calories; protein 18.6g; carbohydrates 51.1g; fat 4.9g; cholesterol 29mg; sodium 719.7mg.

CHAPTER 3: LUNCH

Keto Stuffed Pepper Casserole

Prep:

25 mins

Cook:

47 mins

Total:

1 hr 12 mins

Servings:

8

Yield:

1 casserole

Ingredients

1 head cauliflower, broken into florets

1 pound ground beef

2 cloves garlic, minced

3 green bell peppers, chopped

Italian seasoning

½ cup onion, chopped

¾ cup beef broth

1 teaspoon coconut aminos

2 cups shredded Cheddar cheese

1 (14.5 ounce) can diced tomatoes, drained

Directions

1

Preheat oven to 350 degrees F.

2

Place cauliflower in a food processor and pulse into grounds the size of rice grains. Transfer to a large casserole dish.

3

Combine beef, onion, and garlic in a skillet over medium heat; cook and stir until meat is browned and onion is tender, about 5 minutes. Add green bell peppers and Italian seasoning; continue cooking until slightly tender, about 2 minutes.

4

Drain excess moisture from the beef mixture. Add tomatoes and beef broth. Simmer until flavors combine, about 5 minutes. Add mixture to the cauliflower in the casserole dish; mix to combine. Shake coconut aminos over the casserole; top evenly with Cheddar cheese.

5

Bake in the preheated oven until sauce is bubbly, about 35 minutes.

Nutritions

Per Serving: 260 calories; protein 19.2g; carbohydrates 9.8g; fat 16.5g; cholesterol 65.1mg; sodium 389.4mg.

Thai Chicken Sautè

Prep:

15 mins

Cook:

1 hr 45 mins

Total:

2 hrs

Servings:

8

Yield:

2 quarts

Ingredients

1 chicken carcass

10 cups water

¾ cup thinly sliced galangal

2 kaffir lime leaves, or to taste

2 chopped Thai chiles

2 cloves peeled garlic

1 shallot, sliced

2 stalks lemon grass, crushed

Directions

1

Place the chicken carcass into a large pot and cover with water. Bring to a boil over high heat, then reduce heat to medium-low, and simmer for 5 minutes. Drain, and rinse the carcass under running water. Return the carcass to the pot along with the galangal, lime leaves, lemon grass, chile peppers, garlic, and shallot. Pour in 10 cups of water.

2

Return to a boil over high heat, then reduce heat to medium-low. Simmer uncovered for 1 1/2 hours, skimming the foam and fat often. Strain through cheesecloth before using.

Nutritions

Per Serving: 17 calories; protein 0.5g; carbohydrates 4.1g; fat 0.1g; sodium 11.2mg.

Prosciutto Wrapped Chicken

Prep:

35 mins

Cook:

45 mins

Total:

1 hr 20 mins

Servings:

4

Yield:

4 servings

Ingredients

2 tablespoons olive oil, divided
2 shallots, chopped
1 clove garlic, minced
¼ teaspoon salt
¼ teaspoon ground black pepper
¾ cup soft goat cheese
3 dates, chopped
1 teaspoon chopped fresh thyme
1 tablespoon chopped fresh basil
4 large, thin slices of prosciutto
4 skinless, boneless chicken breast halves

Directions

1

Preheat oven to 350 degrees F. Spread 1 tablespoon of olive oil on a baking sheet, and set aside.

2

Heat 1 tablespoon of olive oil in a skillet over medium heat. Stir in the shallots, and cook until they turn translucent, about 3 minutes. Stir in the garlic, thyme, salt, and pepper; cook and stir an additional 2 minutes. Transfer the shallot mixture to a bowl. Mix in the goat cheese, dates, and basil; stir until well combined.

3

With a sharp knife, cut a 1-inch long slit into the thick side of each chicken breast. Work your fingers into the slit, and expand the slit to form a pocket in the breast meat. With your fingers or a spoon, stuff each chicken breast with about 1/4 cup of the goat cheese mixture. Wipe off any cheese mixture from the outside of the chicken breast, and wrap each breast in a slice of prosciutto so that the pocket opening is covered. Place the chicken breasts, seam sides down, onto the prepared baking sheet.

4

Bake in the preheated oven until the chicken meat is no longer pink and the prosciutto is browned and crisp, about 40 minutes. Turn the chicken breasts over after 20 minutes.

Nutritions

Per Serving: 402 calories; protein 35.6g; carbohydrates 10.4g; fat 24g; cholesterol 105.5mg; sodium 530.2mg.

Low-Carb Chicken and Mushroom Soup

Prep:

20 mins

Cook:

38 mins

Total:

58 mins

Servings:

6

Yield:

6 servings

Ingredients

1 cooked chicken breast, cubed

1 ½ pounds fresh mushrooms, sliced

1 small white onion, finely chopped

3 cloves garlic, finely chopped

3 cups chicken stock

3 tablespoons chopped fresh tarragon, divided

salt and freshly ground black pepper to taste

½ cup butter

2 cups heavy whipping cream

Directions

1

Melt butter in a Dutch oven over medium-high heat. Add chicken; saute until lightly browned, about 3 minutes. Add onion and garlic; saute until softened, about 5 minutes. Stir in mushrooms; saute until tender, 5 to 10 minutes. Pour in chicken stock and 2 tablespoons tarragon; reduce heat to low. Season with salt. Cover and simmer soup until flavors are combined, about 25 minutes.

2

Stir cream into the soup; cook until heated through but not boiling. Serve soup with pepper and the remaining tarragon on top.

Nutritions

Per Serving: 531 calories; protein 15.3g; carbohydrates 8.2g; fat 50.2g; cholesterol 179.2mg; sodium 539.8mg.

Sloppy Joes

Prep:

20 mins

Cook:

25 mins

Total:

45 mins

Servings:

5

Yield:

5 sandwiches

Ingredients

1 ½ pounds lean ground beef

1 yellow onion, chopped

1 red bell pepper, chopped

1 ½ cups ketchup

3 tablespoons apple cider vinegar

3 tablespoons Worcestershire sauce

3 tablespoons brown sugar

sea salt and ground black pepper to taste

3 tablespoons yellow mustard

2 tablespoons grated Parmesan cheese

5 large hamburger buns, toasted

3 tablespoons hickory flavored barbecue sauce

Directions

1

Cook the ground beef in a large skillet over medium heat until completely browned, 5 to 7 minutes. Add the onion and bell pepper, season with sea salt and black pepper, and cook until vegetables soften, about 8 minutes.

2

Stir in the ketchup, vinegar, Worcestershire sauce, brown sugar, mustard, and barbeque sauce. Reduce heat to low and simmer the mixture until thickened, about 10 minutes. Add Parmesan cheese and serve on toasted hamburger buns.

Nutritions

Per Serving: 530 calories; protein 29.6g; carbohydrates 59.4g; fat 19.5g; cholesterol 84.5mg; sodium 1531.4mg.

Pork Stew

Prep:

15 mins

Cook:

2 hrs

Total:

2 hrs 15 mins

Servings:

4

Yield:

4 servings

Ingredients

2 ½ pounds pork shoulder, cut into 2-inch chunks

¼ cup chicken broth

salt and freshly ground black pepper to taste

2 tablespoons vegetable oil

1 large yellow onion, chopped

2 tablespoons apple cider vinegar

½ cup apple cider or apple juice

2 tablespoons Dijon mustard

1 tablespoon prepared horseradish

3 cloves minced garlic

1 ¼ cups heavy cream

1 stalk celery, sliced

1 cup sliced carrots

4 sage leaves

2 sprigs thyme

1 dried bay leaf

2 small sprigs fresh rosemary

1 pinch cayenne pepper

½ cup green peas, fresh or frozen

¼ cup matchstick-cut apple strips

1 tablespoon chopped fresh chives

Directions

1

Season pork chunks generously with salt and pepper. Toss to distribute seasonings evenly.

2

Heat vegetable oil in pot over high heat. Brown pork in batches so meat isn't crowded, about 7 minutes total time per batch. Transfer pork to a plate. Cook onions in same pot; cook and stir until they start to turn translucent and edges get brown, 3 or 4 minutes. Add garlic; cook 1 minute. Stir in apple cider and apple cider vinegar.

3

Raise heat to high. Stir in mustard and horseradish. Transfer browned pork pieces back to pot, along with accumulated juices. Pour in cream and chicken broth to cover. Add sage, thyme, rosemary, and bay leaf. Season with a pinch of salt. Bring to a simmer; reduce heat, cover, and simmer on low for 30 minutes. Add celery, carrots, black pepper and cayenne.

4

Simmer uncovered on low until meat is tender, about 1 hour. Add green peas. Simmer another 10 minutes. Optional: for a thicker sauce, raise heat and simmer until sauce is reduced, 6 to 8 minutes.

5

Garnish individual servings with apple strips and chopped fresh chives.

Nutritions

Per Serving: 760 calories; protein 32.5g; carbohydrates 19.6g; fat 61.2g; cholesterol 213.8mg; sodium 446.5mg.

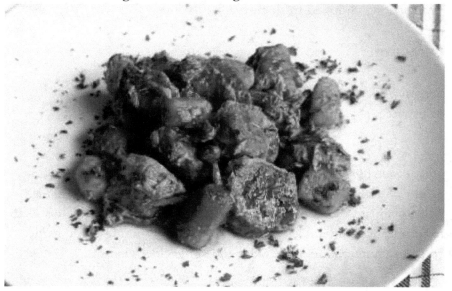

Oven-Roasted Spare Ribs

Prep:

15 mins

Cook:

2 hrs 20 mins

Total:

2 hrs 35 mins

Servings:

4

Yield:

4 servings

Ingredients

1 teaspoon vegetable oil

½ teaspoon dry mustard

½ cup chopped onions

¾ cup chili sauce

½ cup beer

¼ cup honey

2 cloves minced garlic

3 ½ pounds country style pork ribs

2 tablespoons Worcestershire sauce

Directions

1

Heat oil in a saucepan over medium-high heat. Cook and stir onions and garlic in hot oil until fragrant and softened, 4 to 6 minutes.

2

Stir chili sauce, beer, honey, Worcestershire sauce, and dry mustard into onion mixture; bring to a boil, reduce heat to low, and simmer until sauce thickens and flavors develop, 20 minutes.

3

Preheat oven to 350 degrees F.

4

Bake ribs in a baking dish in the preheated oven for 1 hour. Spread sauce over ribs and return to oven; bake until sauce bubbles and ribs are tender, 1 hour.

Nutritions

Per Serving: 634 calories; protein 47.9g; carbohydrates 35.5g; fat 32.2g; cholesterol 178.7mg; sodium 871.5mg.

Carrot Casserole

Prep:

15 mins

Cook:

30 mins

Total:

45 mins

Servings:

6

Yield:

6 servings

Ingredients

5 cups sliced carrots

3 tablespoons butter

1 onion, chopped

1 (10.75 ounce) can condensed cream of celery soup

salt and pepper to taste

½ cup cubed processed cheese

2 cups seasoned croutons

⅓ cup melted butter

Directions

1

Preheat oven to 350 degrees F. Grease a 2 quart casserole dish.

2

Bring a pot of water to a boil. Add carrots and cook until tender but still firm, about 8 minutes; drain.

3

Melt 3 tablespoons butter in a medium saucepan. Saute onions and stir in soup, salt, pepper and cheese. Stir in cooked carrots. Transfer mixture to prepared dish.

4

Toss croutons with 1/3 cup melted butter; scatter over casserole.

5

Bake in preheated oven for 20 to 30 minutes, or until heated through.

Nutritions

Per Serving: 331 calories; protein 6g; carbohydrates 23.1g; fat 24.6g; cholesterol 60.7mg; sodium 909.3mg.

Grilled Spicy Shrimp

Prep:

5 mins

Cook:

5 mins

Total:

10 mins

Servings:

4

Yield:

4 servings

Ingredients

1 pound peeled and deveined shrimp

1 teaspoon smoked paprika

½ teaspoon garlic powder

½ teaspoon onion powder

¼ cup Sriracha chile sauce

½ teaspoon ground cumin

½ teaspoon chili powder

Directions

1

Preheat an outdoor grill for medium-high heat and lightly oil the grate.

2

Put shrimp in a large bowl; add chile sauce, paprika, garlic powder, onion powder, chili powder, and cumin and toss to coat.

3

Place shrimp onto the preheated grill using large tongs and cook until they are bright pink on the outside and the meat is no longer transparent in the center, 3 to 4 minutes.

Nutritions

Per Serving: 101 calories; protein 18.8g; carbohydrates 2.6g; fat 1.1g; cholesterol 172.6mg; sodium 837.4mg.

CHAPTER 4: DINNER

Lemony Grilled Calamari

Prep:

15 mins

Cook:

5 mins

Total:

20 mins

Servings:

10

Yield:

10 appetizer servings

Ingredients

3 cups vegetable oil

¼ cup all-purpose flour

1 teaspoon salt

1 teaspoon dried oregano

½ teaspoon ground black pepper

12 squid, cleaned and sliced into rings

1 lemon - cut into wedges, for garnish

Directions

1

Preheat oil in a heavy, deep frying pan or pot. Oil should be heated to 365 degrees F (180 degrees C).

2

In a medium size mixing bowl mix together flour, salt, oregano and black pepper. Dredge squid through flour and spice mixture.

3

Place squid in oil for 2 to 3 minutes or until light brown. Beware of overcooking, squid will be tough if overcooked. Dry squid on paper towels. Serve with wedges of lemon.

Nutrition

Per Serving: 642 calories; protein 8g; carbohydrates 5.2g; fat 66.7g; cholesterol 111.8mg; sodium 254.1mg.

Tilapia en Papillote

Prep:

25 mins

Cook:

15 mins

Total:

40 mins

Servings:

4

Yield:

4 fillets

Ingredients

4 (4 ounce) fillets tilapia

salt and ground black pepper to taste

1 large tomato, chopped

3 cloves garlic, finely chopped

4 fresh basil leaves, chopped

1 ½ teaspoons capers, drained

4 teaspoons lemon juice

¼ cup butter, divided

1 cup white wine

1 tablespoon butter, or as needed

Directions

1

Preheat oven to 350 degrees F (175 degrees C). Butter a baking sheet so that the bottoms of the packets will brown when baked.

2

Prepare 4 sheets of parchment paper by folding each sheet in half and placing a tilapia fillet centered onto one side of the fold of each sheet. Season the tilapia with salt and black pepper. Top the fillets with equal amounts of tomato, garlic, basil, and capers. Sprinkle lemon juice over the fillets. Place 1 tablespoon butter atop the fish. Drizzle white wine over the fillets.

3

Roll up the sides of the paper first, then the top, leaving 1/2-inch space along one edge; fold to seal. Grease the bottoms of the packets with 1 tablespoon butter and arrange on the baking sheet.

4

Bake in preheated oven until the fish flakes easily with a fork, 15 to 20 minutes.

Nutrition

Per Serving: 303 calories; protein 23.7g; carbohydrates 4.7g; fat 16g; cholesterol 79.1mg; sodium 189.6mg.

Pork Osso Bucco

Prep:

10 mins

Cook:

1 hr 50 mins

Total:

2 hrs

Servings:

2

Yield:

2 servings

Ingredients

2 tablespoons olive oil

1 onion, chopped

3 cloves garlic, chopped

1 pound beef shank

¼ teaspoon dried thyme

¼ teaspoon dried oregano

¼ teaspoon dried rosemary

¼ teaspoon dried marjoram

1 (16 ounce) can diced tomatoes

1 (6 ounce) can tomato paste

water

1 tablespoon lemon zest

1 teaspoon sea salt

½ teaspoon coarsely ground black pepper

Directions

1

Heat olive oil in a large saucepan over medium heat. Add onion and garlic; cook and stir until softened, about 5 minutes. Transfer to a plate. Increase heat to medium-high. Add beef shank and cook until browned, about 5 minutes per side. Return onion and garlic to the pan. Sprinkle thyme, oregano, rosemary, and marjoram over beef.

2

Pour tomatoes and tomato paste into the pan. Fill the empty tomato paste can with water and pour into the pan. Stir in lemon zest, salt, and black pepper. Bring to a boil; reduce heat to low and simmer, covered, until beef is very tender, 1 1/2 to 2 hours.

Nutrition

Per Serving: 520 calories; protein 36.8g; carbohydrates 32.7g; fat 28.9g; cholesterol 79.2mg; sodium 1931.1mg.

Adobo Beef Fajitas

Prep:

15 mins

Cook:

15 mins

Additional:

4 hrs

Total:

4 hrs 30 mins

Servings:

4

Yield:

4 servings

Ingredients

¼ cup olive oil

1 lime, juiced

3 tablespoons chopped fresh cilantro

2 tablespoons finely chopped onion

3 cloves garlic, finely chopped

1 ½ teaspoons ground cumin

1 teaspoon salt

1 teaspoon ground black pepper

2 (8 ounce) boneless New York strip steaks, cut into thin strips

8 (6 inch) white corn tortillas, or more as needed

1 (8 ounce) jar salsa

1 (8 ounce) package shredded Mexican cheese blend

Directions

1

Whisk olive oil, lime juice, cilantro, onion, garlic, cumin, salt, and black pepper in a bowl, and pour into a resealable plastic bag. Add steak strips, coat with the marinade, squeeze out excess air, and seal bag. Marinate in the refrigerator for 4 hours to overnight.

2

Heat a large skillet over medium heat; cook and stir beef in hot skillet until all liquid is absorbed, 15 to 20 minutes.

3

Serve cooked beef with tortillas, salsa and Mexican cheese blend.

Nutrition

Per Serving: 699 calories; protein 49.8g; carbohydrates 31.3g; fat 42.3g; cholesterol 120.6mg; sodium 1450.5mg.

Mashed Cauliflower

Prep:

10 mins

Cook:

45 mins

Total:

55 mins

Servings:

4

Yield:

4 servings

Ingredients

1 head cauliflower, cut into florets
2 tablespoons butter
½ cup milk
½ cup sour cream
1 cup Italian-seasoned bread crumbs
salt and ground black pepper to taste

Directions

1

Preheat the oven to 375 degrees F (190 degrees C).

2

Bring a large pot of water to a boil. Cook cauliflower in the boiling water until tender, about 10 minutes; drain and set aside.

3

Melt butter in the same pot over medium heat. Stir cauliflower, milk, and sour cream into melted butter.

4

Mash cauliflower in the pot using a hand blender until creamy.

5

Transfer cauliflower mixture to a baking dish; evenly cover with bread crumbs and season with salt and black pepper.

6

Baking in the preheated oven until bread crumbs are lightly browned, about 30 minutes.

Nutrition

Per Serving: 274 calories; protein 8.8g; carbohydrates 30.3g; fat 14g; cholesterol 30.4mg; sodium 541.8mg.

Sesame Dipping Sauce

Prep:

10 mins

Cook:

5 mins

Total:

15 mins

Servings:

56

Yield:

7 cups

Ingredients

1 tablespoon olive oil

2 tablespoons minced garlic

4 ½ teaspoons red pepper flakes

2 tablespoons minced fresh ginger root

3 cups soy sauce

3 cups honey

1 cup orange juice

1 tablespoon sesame oil

½ lime, juiced

1 tablespoon sesame seeds

Directions

1

Heat the olive oil in a large skillet over medium heat; cook and stir the garlic and red pepper flakes in the hot oil until fragrant, 2 to 3 minutes.

Add the ginger, soy sauce, honey, orange juice, sesame oil, lime juice, and sesame seeds; stir. Cook until heated, 2 to 3 minutes more.

Nutrition

Per Serving: 71 calories; protein 1g; carbohydrates 16.8g; fat 0.6g; sodium 774mg.

Seitan and Cauliflower

Prep:

20 mins

Cook:

20 mins

Total:

40 mins

Servings:

2

Yield:

2 servings

Ingredients

1 tablespoon vegetable oil

1 (8 ounce) package seitan, sliced

1 ½ teaspoons vegetable oil

½ cup mushrooms, cut into bite-size pieces, or to taste

¼ cup all-purpose flour

1 cup water, or as needed

2 cubes vegetable bouillon

1 pinch cayenne pepper, or to taste (Optional)

1 pinch dried rosemary, or to taste (Optional)

1 pinch dried thyme, or to taste (Optional)

1 small head cauliflower, cut into bite-size pieces

Directions

1

Heat 1 tablespoon oil in a skillet over medium-high heat; saute seitan until cooked through and browned, about 5 minutes. Remove skillet from heat and cover with a lid.

2

Heat 1 1/2 teaspoons vegetable oil in a small saucepan over medium-high heat; saute mushrooms until lightly browned, about 3 minutes. Whisk flour into mushroom mixture using a fork until mushrooms are coated, 2 to 3 minutes.

3

Slowly pour water into mushroom-flour mixture while constantly stirring with a fork until smooth; add bouillon cubes. Decrease heat to medium-low and continue stirring until bouillon is dissolved and gravy is smooth, 5 to 10 minutes more. Season gravy with cayenne pepper, rosemary, and thyme.

4

Mix cauliflower into seitan; cook and stir over medium heat until cauliflower is slightly softened, 3 to 5 minutes. Add gravy; bring to a boil, reduce heat, cover skillet, and simmer, stirring occasionally, until seitan is softened, 7 to 10 minutes.

Nutrition

Per Serving: 347 calories; protein 30.8g; carbohydrates 30.4g; fat 12.7g; sodium 371.2mg.

Baked Maple Glazed Ribs

Prep:

20 mins

Cook:

2 hrs

Total:

2 hrs 20 mins

Servings:

6

Yield:

6 servings

Ingredients

3 pounds pork spareribs, cut into serving size pieces
1 cup pure maple syrup
3 tablespoons ketchup
2 tablespoons soy sauce
1 tablespoon Dijon mustard
1 clove garlic, minced
1 tablespoon Worcestershire sauce
1 teaspoon curry powder
2 green onions, minced
1 tablespoon toasted sesame seeds
3 tablespoons frozen orange juice concentrate

Directions

1

Preheat oven to 350 degrees F. Place ribs meat side up on a rack in a 9x13 inch roasting pan. Cover pan tightly with foil. Bake for 1 1/4 hours.

2

In a saucepan over medium heat, combine maple syrup, orange juice concentrate, ketchup, soy sauce, mustard and Worcestershire sauce. Stir in curry powder, garlic and green onions. Simmer for 15-16 minutes, stirring occasionally.

3

Remove ribs from roasting pan, remove rack, and drain excess fat and drippings. Return ribs to pan, cover with sauce, and bake uncovered for 35 minutes, basting occasionally. Sprinkle with sesame seeds just before serving.

Nutrition

Per Serving: 806 calories; protein 36.2g; carbohydrates 43.1g; fat 54g; cholesterol 181.4mg; sodium 664.4mg.

Creamy Shrimp Shirataki Noodles

Prep:

15 mins

Cook:

5 mins

Total:

20 mins

Servings:

2

Yield:

2 servings

Ingredients

1 (3 ounce) package ramen noodles (flavor packet discarded)
2 tablespoons chopped dry-roasted peanuts
8 ounces frozen cooked shrimp, thawed
½ cup shredded carrot
½ cup thinly bias-sliced celery
⅓ cup bottled chile-lime vinaigrette
½ cup julienned red bell pepper
2 sprigs fresh mint

Directions

1

Cook ramen according to package directions. Drain in a colander under cold running water until cool; drain again.

2

Toss together ramen, shrimp, bell pepper, carrot, celery, and vinaigrette in a bowl. Top servings with peanuts, mint, and black pepper. Serve cold.

Nutrition

Per Serving: 299 calories; protein 26.9g; carbohydrates 16.6g; fat 13.9g; cholesterol 218.4mg; sodium 866.4mg.

Hot Sausage Pot

Prep:

30 mins

Cook:

1 hr

Total:

1 hr 30 mins

Servings:

6

Yield:

6 servings

Ingredients

1 (16 ounce) package spicy ground pork sausage

1 (12 fluid ounce) can beer

2 cups chicken broth

6 large potatoes, peeled and chopped

1 medium red bell pepper, chopped

1 medium yellow bell pepper, chopped

1 large sweet onion, chopped

1 large red onion, chopped

1 jalapeno pepper, finely chopped

1 medium green bell pepper, chopped

1 habanero pepper, seeded and chopped

¼ cup chopped green onions

2 cloves garlic, peeled and chopped

salt and pepper to taste

1 red chile peppers, seeded and chopped

Directions

1

Preheat oven to 350 degrees F.

2

In a large, deep skillet over medium high heat, cook sausage in the beer until evenly browned. Drain, and set aside.

3

In a large baking dish, mix sausage, potatoes, green bell pepper, red bell pepper, yellow bell pepper, sweet onion, red onion, jalapeno pepper, habanero pepper, red chile pepper, green onions, and garlic. Season with salt and pepper. Stir in chicken broth.

4

Cover, and bake in the preheated oven 1 hour, or until all vegetables are tender.

Nutrition

Per Serving: 668 calories; protein 18g; carbohydrates 76.9g; fat 31.1g; cholesterol 51.5mg; sodium 535.1mg.

CHAPTER 5: APPETIZER, SNACKS & SIDE DISHES

Baba Ghanoush

Prep:

5 mins

Cook:

40 mins

Additional:

3 hrs

Total:

3 hrs 45 mins

Servings:

12

Yield:

1 1/2 cups

Ingredients

1 eggplant
¼ cup lemon juice
¼ cup tahini
2 tablespoons sesame seeds
2 cloves garlic, minced
salt and pepper to taste
1 ½ tablespoons olive oil

Directions

1

Preheat oven to 400 degrees F (200 degrees C). Lightly grease a baking sheet.

2

Place eggplant on baking sheet, and make holes in the skin with a fork. Roast it for 30 to 40 minutes, turning occasionally, or until soft. Remove from oven, and place into a large bowl of cold water. Remove from water, and peel skin off.

3

Place eggplant, lemon juice, tahini, sesame seeds, and garlic in an electric blender, and puree. Season with salt and pepper to taste. Transfer eggplant mixture to a medium size mixing bowl, and slowly mix in olive oil. Refrigerate for 3 hours before serving.

Nutrition

Per Serving: 66 calories; protein 1.6g; carbohydrates 4.6g; fat 5.2g; sodium 7mg.

Paprika & Dill Deviled Eggs

Prep:

15 mins

Cook:

15 mins

Additional:

10 mins

Total:

40 mins

Servings:

12

Yield:

24 deviled eggs

Ingredients

12 large eggs

6 tablespoons mayonnaise

2 tablespoons sweet relish

4 teaspoons dried dill weed

1 teaspoon mustard

¼ teaspoon salt

¼ teaspoon ground black pepper

1 teaspoon smoked paprika

Directions

1

Place eggs in a saucepan and cover with water. Bring to a boil, remove from heat, and let eggs stand in hot water for 10 to 12 minutes.

2

While eggs are cooking, combine mayonnaise, relish, dill, mustard, salt, and pepper in a medium mixing bowl.

3

Remove eggs from hot water, cool under cold running water, and peel. Halve eggs lengthwise; remove yolks and add to mayonnaise mixture. Mix well. Scoop mixture into a piping bag or plastic baggie. Place in the refrigerator until more firm, 10 to 15 minutes.

4

Pipe the chilled mixture into the emptied and halved eggs. Sprinkle paprika on top of each egg. Serve immediately or refrigerate for up to 7 days.

Nutrition

Per Serving: 126 calories; protein 6.5g; carbohydrates 1.8g; fat 10.5g; cholesterol 188.6mg; sodium 183.5mg.

All Seed Flapjacks

Prep:

15 mins

Cook:

15 mins

Total:

30 mins

Servings:

8

Yield:

8 servings

Ingredients

½ cup butter

3 tablespoons white sugar

2 tablespoons golden syrup

2 cups rolled oats

5 tablespoons raisins (Optional)

1 (5 ounce) milk chocolate, melted (Optional)

Directions

1

Preheat the oven to 350 degrees F (175 degrees C). Lightly butter a baking pan.

2

Combine butter, sugar, and golden syrup in a saucepan over low heat. Mix until butter has melted and sugar has dissolved. Remove from heat. Add 2 cups oats and raisins. Mix until oats are well coated. Pour mixture into the prepared pan; flatten down with the back of a spoon.

3
Bake in the preheated oven until golden brown on top, 10 to 20 minutes. Let flapjack cool.

4
Melt chocolate in a microwave-safe glass or ceramic bowl in 15-second intervals, stirring after each interval, 1 to 3 minutes. Pour over the cooled flapjack. Let cool until chocolate is set.

Nutrition
Per Serving: 330 calories; protein 4.4g; carbohydrates 38.5g; fat 18.4g; cholesterol 34.8mg; sodium 101.6mg.

CHAPTER 6: VEGAN & VEGETARIAN

Key Lime Thyme Pie

Prep:

15 mins

Cook:

10 mins

Total:

25 mins

Servings:

8

Yield:

1 pie

Ingredients

Crust:
2 cups gluten-free graham crackers, blended
¼ cup vegan butter, melted
Sweetened Condensed Milk:
2 (11 ounce) bottles So Delicious® Culinary Coconut Milk
1 pinch salt
¼ teaspoon vanilla extract
2 cups powdered sugar

Filling:
2 tablespoons organic cane sugar
¾ cup key lime juice, or to taste
1 lime, zested
1 (9 ounce) tub So Delicious® Dairy Free CocoWhip

Topping:
Candied thyme, for garnish (see directions)

Directions

1

For the crust, blend an 8 oz. box of gluten-free graham crackers to make 2 cups of crumbs. Stir in the melted vegan butter until combined.

2

Pat the mixture into the bottom of a standard pie dish or a spring form, oiled and sides lined with parchment paper. Use the bottom of a drinking glass to help press the mixture flat to the bottom.

3

Bake at 350 degrees for 8-10 minutes.

4

Dairy-free Sweetened Condensed Milk: In a small/medium size saucepan pour in the bottles of coconut culinary milk and bring to a low boil. Allow to boil for 5 minutes while whisking continuously.

5

Lower the heat bringing the milk to a simmer. Add in the powdered sugar and continue to whisk until the sugar has fully dissolved. Add thyme sprigs, salt and vanilla (if using) and allow to simmer until the mixture has reduced by half - about 30-40 minutes. Remove sprigs from milk.

6

Candied Thyme Garnish: Create a simple syrup by bringing equal parts water and organic cane syrup to a boil and simmering until the sugar is dissolved. Once the mixture has cooled completely, dip fresh sprigs of thyme into it and lay them onto parchment paper. Sprinkle with sugar.

7

For the Filling:

8

Add the key lime juice to the Sweetened Condensed Milk with thyme, to taste.

9

Fold the CocoWhip in to the mixture and add lime zest to taste.

10

Add the filling to the crust, lightly cover and freeze for at least 2 hours or overnight.

11

Garnish with key lime slices and sprigs of candied thyme.

Nutrition

Per Serving: 433 calories; protein 2.5g; carbohydrates 59.8g; fat 22.7g; sodium 202.1mg.

Tofu Radish Bowls

Prep:

10 mins

Total:

10 mins

Servings:

4

Yield:

1 large bowl

Ingredients

3 green onions, chopped

2 tablespoons soy sauce

2 tablespoons toasted sesame seeds

1 ½ teaspoons Korean chile pepper powder

1 teaspoon white sugar

½ teaspoon toasted Asian sesame oil

1 ½ cups steamed Japanese rice

½ cucumber - peeled, seeded, and chopped

1 (12 ounce) package tofu, sliced

½ head of romaine lettuce (heart only), torn into bite-size pieces

Directions

1

Mix green onions, soy sauce, sesame seeds, Korean red pepper powder, sugar, and sesame oil together in a bowl until evenly combined.

2

Place rice in a serving bowl. Toss lettuce and cucumber together and place onto rice. Arrange tofu over lettuce and cucumber. Drizzle sesame mixture over tofu to taste.

Nutrition

Per Serving: 198 calories; protein 10.4g; carbohydrates 23.7g; fat 7.2g; sodium 471.8mg.

Pasta with Alfredo Sauce

Prep:

10 mins

Cook:

10 mins

Total:

20 mins

Servings:

4

Yield:

4 servings

Ingredients

¼ cup butter

1 ½ cups freshly grated Parmesan cheese

¼ cup chopped fresh parsley

1 cup heavy cream

1 clove garlic, crushed

Directions

1

Melt butter in a medium saucepan over medium low heat. Add cream and simmer for 5 minutes, then add garlic and cheese and whisk quickly, heating through. Stir in parsley and serve.

Nutrition

Per Serving: 439 calories; protein 13g; carbohydrates 3.4g; fat 42.1g; cholesterol 138.4mg; sodium 565.3mg.

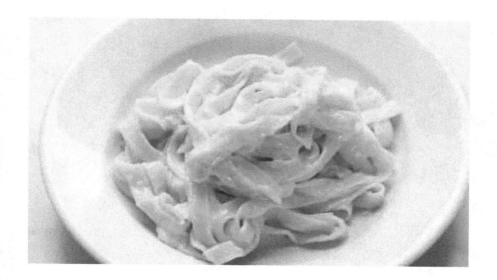

Aromatic Chinese Cabbage

Prep:

15 mins

Cook:

10 mins

Total:

25 mins

Servings:

12

Yield:

12 servings

Ingredients

1 (3 ounce) package ramen noodles, crushed

1 bunch green onions, chopped

½ cup white sugar

½ cup vegetable oil

¼ cup cider vinegar

10 ounces cashew pieces

1 (16 ounce) package shredded coleslaw mix

1 tablespoon soy sauce

Directions

1

In a preheated 350 degree F oven, toast the crushed noodles and nuts until golden brown.

2

In a large bowl, combine the coleslaw, green onions, toasted ramen noodles and cashews.

3

To prepare the dressing, whisk together the sugar, oil, vinegar and soy sauce. Pour the dressing over the salad, toss and serve.

Nutrition

Per Serving: 291 calories; protein 4.6g; carbohydrates 22.8g; fat 21.3g; cholesterol 3mg; sodium 262.9mg.

CHAPTER 7: DESSERTS

Cherry Cobbler

Prep:

1 hr

Cook:

1 hr

Total:

2 hrs

Servings:

12

Yield:

12 servings

Ingredients

½ cup butter

1 cup all-purpose flour

1 cup white sugar   .

1 cup milk

¾ cup white sugar

1 teaspoon baking powder

1 tablespoon all-purpose flour

2 cups pitted sour cherries

Directions

1

Preheat the oven to 350 degrees F. Place the butter in a 9x13 inch baking dish, and place in the oven to melt while the oven is preheating. Remove as soon as butter has melted, about 5 minutes.

2

In a medium bowl, stir together 1 cup of flour, 1 cup of sugar, and baking powder. Mix in the milk until well blended, then pour the batter into the pan over the butter. Do not stir.

3

Rinse out the bowl from the batter, and dry. Place cherries into the bowl, and toss with the remaining 3/4 cup of sugar and 1 tablespoon of flour. Distribute the cherry mixture evenly over the batter. Do not stir.

4

Bake for 50 to 60 minutes in the preheated oven, until golden brown. A toothpick inserted into the cobber should come out clean.

Nutrition

Per Serving: 244 calories; protein 2.2g; carbohydrates 41.8g; fat 8.3g; cholesterol 22mg; sodium 93.8mg.

Chocolate and Nuts

Prep:

10 mins

Cook:

2 hrs

Total:

2 hrs 10 mins

Servings:

60

Yield:

60 servings

Ingredients

2 pounds skinless, salted peanuts
1 (12 ounce) package milk chocolate chips
1 (4 ounce) package sweet baking chocolate (such as Baker's German's Sweet Chocolate®), broken into pieces
24 ounces white almond bar, broken into pieces

Directions

1

Pour peanuts into your slow cooker. Layer sweet baking chocolate over the peanuts. Spread milk chocolate chips onto the baking chocolate. Finish with a layer of white almond bar pieces.

2

Cook on Low for 2 hours before stirring to mix evenly.

3

Line baking sheets with waxed paper or baking parchment. Drop spoonfuls of the peanut mixture onto the prepared baking sheets. Set aside until the candies harden. Store covered in a cool place.

Nutrition

Per Serving: 181 calories; protein 5g; carbohydrates 13.1g; fat 14.4g; cholesterol 1.9mg; sodium 132.9mg.

Chocolate Bar Hot Chocolate

Prep:

5 mins

Cook:

5 mins

Total:

10 mins

Servings:

1

Yield:

1 serving

Ingredients

⅔ cup milk

1 (1.55 ounce) bar milk chocolate candy bar, chopped

Directions

1

Place chocolate pieces in a saucepan over medium-low heat; add milk and whisk constantly until chocolate is melted and well blended, about 5 minutes. Whisk in cinnamon. Remove from heat; add more milk if desired. Serve in a mug.

Nutrition

Per Serving: 319 calories; protein 8.8g; carbohydrates 34.6g; fat 16.3g; cholesterol 23.1mg; sodium 101.6mg.

Coconut Macaroon

Servings:
24
Yield:
4 dozen

Ingredients

5 ½ cups flaked coconut
2 teaspoons vanilla extract
1 ½ teaspoons almond extract
1 (14 ounce) can sweetened condensed milk

Directions
1
Preheat oven to 350 degrees F.

2
In large mixing bowl, combine coconut, sweetened condensed milk and extracts; mix well.

3
Drop by rounded teaspoonfuls onto aluminum foil-lined and generously greased baking sheets. Bake 8 to 10 minutes or until lightly browned around the edges. Immediately remove from baking sheets. Store loosely covered at room temperature.

Nutrition
Per Serving: 132 calories; protein 1.8g; carbohydrates 17.7g; fat 6.2g; cholesterol 5.6mg; sodium 69.1mg.

Almond Ice Cream

Prep:

40 mins

Additional:

12 hrs

Total:

12 hrs 40 mins

Servings:

6

Yield:

6 servings

Ingredients

2 (14 ounce) cans full-fat coconut milk, chilled overnight

¼ cup tahini

1 teaspoon almond extract

5 pitted dates, soaked in hot water for 30 minutes and drained

¼ cup sliced almonds

Directions

1

Freeze the base of your ice cream maker for at least 12 hours.

2

Combine coconut milk, 1/2 cup strawberries, tahini, dates, and almond extract in a high-speed blender. Blend until strawberries are broken down and mixture is combined, about 1 minute. Pour mixture into an ice cream maker and churn according to manufacturer's directions, 5 to 9 minutes.

3

As mixture starts to thicken, add remaining 1/2 strawberries and sliced almonds. Continue mixing until thickened, 10 to 20 minutes more.

4

Serve immediately as soft-serve ice cream garnished with additional strawberries and sesame seeds. Alternatively, place ice cream in the freezer for 1 to 2 hours to firm up.

Nutrition

Per Serving: 428 calories; protein 6.2g; carbohydrates 27.2g; fat 36.2g; sodium 29.4mg.

White Chocolate Mousse

Prep:

20 mins

Cook:

6 mins

Additional:

6 hrs 30 mins

Total:

6 hrs 56 mins

Servings:

16

Yield:

16 servings

Ingredients

1 (20 ounce) package holiday chocolate sandwich cookies (such as Oreos®), divided

1 ¼ cups milk

1 (.25 ounce) package unflavored gelatin (such as Knox ®)

1 (11 ounce) package white chocolate chips

6 tablespoons butter, melted

¼ cup fresh raspberries, for garnish

1 pint heavy whipping cream

Directions

1

Place 24 cookies in a zip top bag and seal it. Finely crush the cookies with a rolling pin. Transfer cookie crumbs to a mixing bowl. Drizzle melted butter over the crumbs; mix well. Press crumbs on the bottom and up the sides of a 9-inch springform pan, forming a crust.

2

Pour milk into a saucepan. Sprinkle gelatin on the milk; let stand 1 minute. Place pan over low heat; stir milk until gelatin dissolves, about 3 minutes. Add white chocolate chips; stir until melted, about 3 minutes. Refrigerate until mixture is slightly thickened, about 30 minutes.

3

Beat cream in a chilled glass or metal bowl with an electric mixer until soft peaks form.

4

Coarsely break up or chop 24 cookies. Fold cookie pieces and whipped cream into the white chocolate mixture. Spoon into prepared springform pan. Refrigerate 6 hours or overnight.

5

Twist the remaining cookies into 2 rounds each. Garnish cake with cookie halves and fresh raspberries.

Nutrition

Per Serving: 425 calories; protein 4.9g; carbohydrates 37.9g; fat 29.2g; cholesterol 57.8mg; sodium 240.1mg.

Keto Vanilla Ice Cream

Prep:

10 mins

Additional:

3 hrs

Total:

3 hrs 10 mins

Servings:

3

Yield:

3 servings

Ingredients

1 cup heavy whipping cream

¼ teaspoon xanthan gum

2 tablespoons powdered zero-calorie sweetener (such as Swerve®)

1 teaspoon vanilla extract

1 pinch salt

1 tablespoon vodka

Directions

1

Combine cream, sweetener, vodka, vanilla extract, xanthan gum, and salt in a wide-mouth pint-sized jar. Blend cream mixture with an immersion blender in an up-and-down motion until cream has thickened and soft peaks have formed, 60 to 75 seconds. Cover jar and place in the freezer for 3 to 4 hours, stirring every 30 to 40 minutes.

Nutrition

Per Serving: 291 calories; protein 1.6g; carbohydrates 3.2g; fat 29.4g; cholesterol 108.7mg; sodium 91.7mg.

Rum Coconut Candy

Servings:

4

Yield:

4 to 5 servings

Ingredients

1 (12 ounce) package vanilla wafers, crushed
1 cup finely chopped walnuts
1 (14 ounce) can sweetened condensed milk
⅛ cup confectioners' sugar
¼ cup rum
1 ⅓ cups flaked coconut

Directions

1

In a large bowl, combine crumbs, coconut, & nuts. Add sweetened condensed milk & rum; mix well. Chill 4 hours.

2

Shape into 1- inch balls. Roll in sugar. Store in covered container in refrigerator 24 hours before serving.

Nutrition

Per Serving: 1063 calories; protein 16.6g; carbohydrates 133.7g; fat 50.8g; cholesterol 33.3mg; sodium 452.6mg

Hemp Seed Soup

Prep:

20 mins

Cook:

30 mins

Total:

50 mins

Servings:

4

Yield:

4 servings

Ingredients

4 cups water
1 cube vegetable bouillon, or more to taste
¾ cup red lentils
2 bay leaves
¼ pound hemp seeds
½ pound carrots, chopped
¼ pound fresh mushrooms, finely chopped
1 tablespoon olive oil
1 onion, chopped
2 cloves garlic, minced
1 bunch cilantro, chopped
salt and ground black pepper to taste

Directions

1

Bring water to a boil in a large pot and add vegetable bouillon to taste. Add lentils and bay leaves and simmer for 15 minutes. Add carrots, mushrooms, salt, and pepper; continue to simmer.

2

Heat olive oil in a skillet over medium-high heat; saute onion until soft, about 5 minutes. Add garlic and saute until fragrant, 1 to 2 minutes. Stir onion mixture into the soup.

3

Cook and stir hemp seeds in a separate skillet over medium-high heat until toasted and fragrant, 2 to 3 minutes. Stir toasted hemp seeds into soup. Add cilantro and cook 5 minutes more.

Nutrition

Per Serving: 372 calories; protein 21g; carbohydrates 37.7g; fat 16.5g; sodium 100.1mg.

Nutella Brownies

Prep:

15 mins

Cook:

25 mins

Additional:

2 hrs

Total:

2 hrs 40 mins

Servings:

16

Yield:

16 servings

Ingredients

½ cup butter

¼ cup hazelnut liqueur (such as Frangelico®)

¼ teaspoon salt

⅔ cup white sugar

1 cup all-purpose flour, sifted

½ cup unsweetened cocoa powder

⅓ cup brown sugar

2 eggs

1 teaspoon vanilla extract

¼ cup chocolate-hazelnut spread (such as Nutella®)

Directions

1

Preheat oven to 375 degrees F. Grease an 8-inch square baking pan or line with parchment paper.

2

Melt butter, hazelnut liqueur, and chocolate-hazelnut spread together in a small saucepan over medium heat, stirring occasionally, until starting to bubble, about 5 minutes. Remove saucepan from heat and cool slightly.

3

Whisk flour, cocoa powder, and salt together in a bowl.

4

Beat white sugar, brown sugar, eggs, and vanilla extract together in a large bowl using an electric mixer until smooth and creamy; slowly mix in butter mixture until smooth. Stir flour mixture into butter-sugar mixture just until batter is combined; fold in chocolate chips, if using. Pour batter into the prepared pan.

5

Bake in the preheated oven until the top is dry and the edges have started to pull away from the sides of the pan, 20 to 25 minutes. Cool brownies in pan for at least 2 hours before cutting.

Nutrition

Per Serving: 204 calories; protein 2.7g; carbohydrates 27.8g; fat 9.5g; cholesterol 38.5mg; sodium 92.6mg.

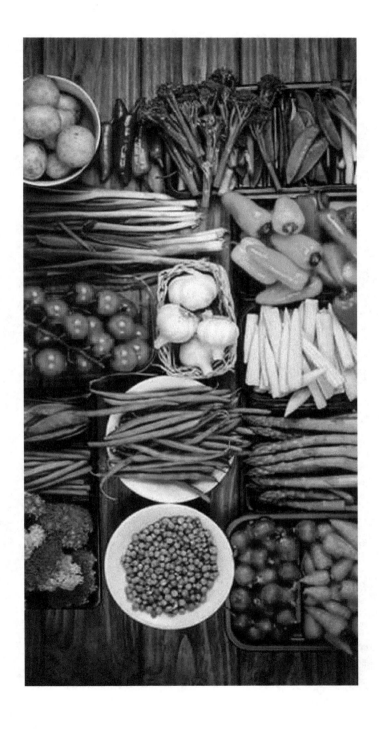

CPSIA information can be obtained
at www.ICGtesting.com
Printed in the USA
BVHW051356270421
605941BV00002B/64